Those Who Care:

A Guided Journal for Past, Present, and Future Caregivers

Tasha M. Livingston

These are my memories from my perspective, and I have tried to represent events as faithfully as possible. This journal does not replace the advice of a medical professional. Consult a physician to confirm all steps and expectations of your loved one's pre-operative and post-operative periods.

Edited By: Nicole Narvaez Manns and Sierra Dean

ISBN: 978-0-578-75564-9

DEDICATION

This journal is dedicated to Rina Kader and Wayne J. Livingston. Rina is my "Sister living in My Mister," the donor who saved my husband's life on October 22, 2018. To my husband, Wayne J. Livingston – God kept you here because you are the example of what the world needs more of. I love you for life!

This Journal Belongs To:

_____

Caregiver For:

_____

Journey Start Date:

_____

CONTENTS

The Purpose and How to Use This Journal:

"Those Who Care" is for the people who love and support transplant patients. No one truly knows what it feels like to be the caregiver of a transplant patient except for others who have been down that same road as well. Over time you realize that you're now a part of a larger community of people who understand where you are coming from and what you've been through.

After going through this experience, it is important for me to tell our story from a caregiver perspective and to shed light on the different seasons of the journey. It is important for me to provide a space for those individuals who have already been, currently are, or are getting ready to be caregivers of a transplant recipient. The transplant process is very tedious, and I found it helpful to chronicle the journey. This journal will guide you with short passages from my personal journey as a caregiver for my husband during his transplant journey.

You'll read small excerpts from each season of our journey, and I have provided you with space to write your own experiences. You will experience an emotional roller coaster as certain milestone date occurs. This is your space to express your thoughts! On a personal note, I did not know anyone who had experienced a transplant journey prior to our experience, and it was important for me to break that cycle by creating this journal. **This is your safe space!**

1 When We First Found Out

My husband Wayne was diagnosed with Primary Sclerosing Cholangitis and Ulcerative Colitis in 2007, about a year and a half before we met. He didn't keep it a secret from me and gave me the choice to either ride this wave with him or not. He was given 7-15 years to live, and at that time a transplant wasn't in the discussions.

In the beginning you'd never know anything was going on with him, but as the years passed, symptoms started to appear, and gradually got worse. My husband Wayne experienced multiple tests, periodic procedures, and scopes. Prior to transplant the biggest scare was when he ended up hospitalized for a week with E-Coli. I honestly didn't know what the outcome of that was going to be, because he was extremely sick with a high fever. He made it through without any additional problems! As you can imagine there were moments of peace and moments of extreme stress. When Wayne was feeling good — he was feeling good, so I was feeling good. Every time he got sick it was a reminder that we were dealing with something we had no control over, and all I could do was pray that it did not progress, and that he would feel better. We spent years of praying that this disease would stay dormant. Wishful thinking you could call it.

Overtime I became a professional back scratcher because his skin was always itching. He often asked me to look in his eyes and confirm if they were still white. I watched as he tried on clothes that were becoming too big as each month passed. I saw him not wanting to do much because he was fatigued and did not want any sympathy from anyone. I spent many moments being asked "Where's Wayne?" at social events — this was when he was beginning to have less and less energy and chose to stay home. He didn't like to go out a ton because his eyes were beginning to show jaundice. Jaundice is a symptom of liver disease and usually the skin and eyes become discolored and yellow. The hardest part of all of this was that few people knew the extent of what he was dealing with. He didn't talk about it to others and in turn, neither did I unless it was with each other or with immediate family. Those who were close to us knew he had liver problems; however, they didn't know the severity of it or that he may one day need a transplant.

Fast forward to when he had just gotten a routine scope. While he was in recovery his physician came out to talk to us and told us that his disease had progressed, and at this point he needed to follow up with his liver specialist. I felt like in this moment we all truly understood how sick he was. My heart dropped because I kind of knew where this was headed, but I was still unwilling to hear it. I was terrified and in denial.

We walked into the doctor's office on April 18, 2018, and the first thing the specialist said to him was: "So have you started looking into the living donor liver transplant option?" Apparently the one and only visit that I didn't attend in February is when the physician first mentioned this, but Wayne didn't know he meant *immediately,* so he never said anything to me. Imagine my horror. This was something we knew was a possibility, but now it was reality, and it was scary as hell. It was at this visit that we found out that he was a lot sicker than we wanted to believe. All of his current symptoms: the itching, the jaundice, and the weight loss had all come full circle.

We both hoped this moment would never happen, but yet it did. I was on the phone with the transplant department before we were even out of our parking space. I clearly remember telling them to test me first so we could get this over with. They took down all of my information, however by the end of the conversation when I told them I would be his caregiver I was advised I would only be considered as a last resort option. If I were a match and donated, we would both need a caregiver 24 hours a day during recovery. As his wife I felt completely helpless because I couldn't save his life. I was angry that we were a few months behind, scared because I knew this could be fatal, sad because I hated seeing my husband having to go through this, happy that there was an option to prolong his life, anxious at the unknown, and ready to get this show on the road. I felt like I didn't have enough time to appropriately process all of these feelings because it was show time. We had to find a donor, and I had to be strong for the both of us.

How did you find out and what were your initial thoughts and actions?

_____

_____

_____

_____

_____

_____

_____

_____

_____

_____

_____

_____

_____

_____

_____

_____

_____

_____

_____

_____

2 Mental & Spiritual Preparation

How exactly do you prepare for something when you have no idea what the outcome is going to be? As a wife I had feelings of "Oh my goodness! My husband is getting ready to undergo this huge procedure." "What if we can't find a donor?" "What if he doesn't make it?" "What is really happening?" "What is HE feeling?" Not to mention the indirect feelings that came as a result of what some of his thoughts were; for example, him not knowing if he was going to live long enough to be transplanted or die waiting! His thoughts/feelings of "What if these are my last days? If so, how do I really want to spend them?" This was TOUGH stuff to process. But it was our reality!

It is a very lonely process and sometimes there are thoughts that you don't feel comfortable sharing with anyone outside of yourself and GOD because you don't want to stress anyone out or feel selfish since you aren't the one physically going through it. But emotionally you are and that is HUGE! I didn't initially share my thoughts with my husband because I especially did not want him to stress even more. He already had enough on his plate. I definitely remember putting on my "I'm okay" mask on for a long while even before we got to this point. I found myself keeping busy in a sales business I was a part of for a few years because it was a good distraction from my reality that I now had to really face. I couldn't always hide how I was feeling. I remember specifically vending at an event with two other people. I was late and I am NEVER late and while there I was totally off my game, unfocused, and stress shopping. I was stressed out and I was beyond scared. But I had to snap out of it and remember that God did not give me a spirit of fear. I had to tap into my faith and understand that we would not be going through this if we weren't going to get through it. God already knew the outcome and it was time for my faith to grow stronger than ever before and prepare for the next steps ahead.

After a visit with one of the physicians on the transplant team, we finally put his story out on social media in June 2018. I felt relieved because at least now, there was nothing hidden, and everyone knew what we were dealing with. We set up a Facebook page with a hashtag of #LivingWithTheLivingstons for others to keep up with the journey. The outpouring of love, prayers, and offers to assist were overwhelming. People that I had gone to school with more than 10 years ago were willing to see if they were a match! We had also attended a Living Donor Liver Transplant Workshop at UPMC (University of Pittsburgh Medical Center), and we met a few more members of the transplant team. I began to feel that everything was going to be just fine and reassured myself that God was ordering our steps. I began to breathe, and my heart began to beat normally again without anxiety.

During this same summer I had attended an event for the company I was working with at the time. One of the activities they had us do was stand up, close our eyes, and envision our ideal day. I vividly remember closing my eyes, and automatically being brought to a space of peace. I saw us waking up in a house full of natural light, getting up having breakfast, and getting ready for our day. We were headed our separate ways only to meet up after and head to a conference to speak about the outcome of his transplant. We were on a stage and he was sharing his testimony with others who needed encouragement. After five minutes we were told to open our eyes, and I had happy tears streaming down my face. I felt like that small activity was God's way of giving me a glimpse of what our post-transplant journey would look like. I held on to this thought the rest of the way because the law of attraction is real, and we were going to manifest this exact scene!

How were you able to prepare for what was to come and what was your mental and emotional state during this time?

_____

_____

_____

_____

_____

_____

_____

_____

_____

_____

_____

_____

_____

_____

_____

_____

_____

_____

_____

_____

_____

_____

_____

_____

_____

_____

_____

_____

_____

_____

_____

_____

_____

_____

_____

_____

_____

_____

_____

_____

3 We Found A Donor

Wayne cuts grass in the warmer weather months and little did he know he wasn't cutting for extra income, but he was cutting grass to save his life. One day he was cutting grass for his client Rina. He had to tell her that he may not be able to finish out the season because he needed a liver transplant. He then found out Rina was just days away from becoming an altruistic donor for children, and just like that she immediately decided she wanted to donate to Wayne. She contacted the department and got all the necessary screening, and we were now able to get Wayne set up for all of his pre-op testing. We couldn't do this previously due to former insurance company policies. I remember being so upset that he couldn't be seen initially, because at that time the two insurance companies decided "not to get along" for lack of a better explanation. I hated that someone could potentially get sicker while waiting just because of paperwork. I was upset that even in the name of life or death, everything seemed to be "just a number." The system goes by a "MELD Score" which stands for Model End Stage Liver Disease, and sometimes you may be sicker than your score reflects, thus affecting your position on the transplant waiting list. For this reason, I was and will always be grateful for the living donor option. It is more flexible and gives the patient the opportunity to get their transplant while they are at an optimal point in their journey. If

18

your doctor has not talked about this option yet please bring it up to them as it just may be the way to save your loved one's life!

I'll never forget the evaluation process. It was two full days of every test you could imagine. This was scary because we didn't know if the tests were going to uncover something else that we didn't know about or something that would delay moving forward with the transplant. Thankfully all was well, and we were able to proceed. A little time passed, and of course I wanted to meet Rina, the woman who would potentially save his life. While at her home Wayne casually asked what her blood type was. "O+" she said. I remember bawling as soon as she said her type, because O+ is what Wayne needed! I knew then that he would be okay, because this was no coincidence! The level of peace I felt leaving her home was priceless. Everything just felt RIGHT!

Fast forward to September 2018 we were laying on the bed, and Wayne got a text message from Rina saying she had been approved to be his donor. I remember the evening like it was yesterday; we looked at each other and our jaws dropped. We sat in silence for a few moments before realizing that this was really happening! After a few months and one simple conversation here was the moment we had been hoping and praying for. Wayne was going to get a liver!

What came next was scary but exciting at the same time — figuring out a day to schedule it. We didn't want to prolong it since we had someone ready and willing. His birthday and the holidays were approaching also! We decided on October 22, 2018 as the surgery date. This gave everyone enough time to get things situated, and he would be able to enjoy his 37th birthday without worry. I remember telling him I wasn't sure what to give him for his birthday, because well, you can't top a new liver.

Think about when you found out there was a donor available, and your loved one was going to get a chance at a new life. How did it happen and what feelings do you recall having? If you are still waiting for a donor, what are you feeling right now?

_____

_____

_____

_____

_____

_____

_____

_____

_____

_____

_____

_____

_____

_____

_____

_____

_____

_____

_____

_____

_____

_____

_____

_____

_____

_____

_____

_____

_____

_____

_____

_____

_____

_____

_____

_____

_____

_____

_____

_____

_____

_____

_____

_____

_____

_____

_____

_____

_____

_____

_____

_____

_____

_____

_____

_____

_____

_____

_____

_____

_____

_____

_____

_____

_____

_____

_____

_____

_____

_____

_____

_____

_____

_____

_____

_____

_____

_____

_____

4 When Things Got Real

I remember the day of the pre-operative appointment as if it were yesterday. This was the date we had to meet with the entire transplant team including the transplant surgeons, the nutritionist, the social worker, hepatologist, pharmacist, and anesthesiologists, just to name a few. It was a long day. When it came time to talk to the surgeons, I asked them to tell me *exactly* what to expect from the time we got to the hospital until after surgery, and I specifically asked them not to sugarcoat anything. I remember taking verbatim notes and I am going to share them below.

My personal notes from the pre-op appointment on what to expect the day of transplant:

- 5 am - arrival to the hospital
- 7:30 am - Wayne will be in a holding area.
- Rina will already be there and possibly in the operating room.
- Around 8-8:30 am - Wayne will be with surgeon #1 for an hour and a half to get ready for surgery ex. IV, tubes, catheter, and ventilator.
- Surgery will start close to 10 am.
- They will close off the end of the bile duct that used to go to the liver.
- The new bile duct will connect directly to the intestines; this should be done by 1-2 pm.

- Wayne's liver will be removed, and he will be temporarily placed on a bypass machine and they will use a bypass cannula to circulate blood to the heart.

- There will be constant communication with surgeon #2.

- The new liver from Rina will have veins lengthened and the veins will come from either the fridge, the old liver, or his leg. (I'll get into the fridge part later in this chapter).

- Both surgeons will work together to get the new liver working; this will take until about 6 pm-7 pm.

- Will there be Tubes? Yes - there will be three of them.

  o One drain next to the liver to keep fluid out of the liver. That will stay in for about 1-2 weeks.

  o One or two skinny tubes will be inserted up through the bile duct connection to allow scar tissue to heal around the tube. These will be removed in 2-3 months.

  o One little wire will have a sensor on the end that will sit on the main blood vessel that will be carrying blood into the liver. It will be plugged into a box to hear the blood flowing into the artery. This will stay in about five days.

- The surgeon will come out and talk to the family.

- Scans will be done afterwards to ensure everything is working correctly.

- Wayne will spend the night in intensive care (ICU) to be closely monitored.

- It is expected he will be out of bed the next day, up and walking; getting physical therapy to bounce back quickly.

- They will watch for problems such as bleeding. They will ensure the liver is working properly. They will ensure there are no blood clots. They will look at all of the blood vessels the next day and make sure the bile duct tube heals well. At this point, he will be moved to a regular room.

Out of all of this, at the time my immediate main concern was the fridge veins. It was explained to me that there was no way of knowing the health of the veins in terms of if they came from a high-risk patient with a communicable disease. I was reassured that tests would be done after the surgery to confirm, and if there was anything identified then there would be treatment available. This blew my mind in addition to the fact that there wasn't a guarantee there would be veins readily available. The other option would have been an additional procedure to remove veins from his legs. I did not feel comfortable with this option either. The most horrific choice to me was the option of needing to use the veins from his original liver. I was thinking, "Why is this even a thing?" If the liver is bad; we don't want the veins from it either! I had to pray and have faith that there would be GOOD veins available for use and then just leave it alone. At this point there was nothing I could do but the same thing I had been doing for the past few years - PRAY! This was a LOT to take in, but having the information upfront helped to calm my nerves, and I knew exactly what my husband was getting ready to endure. Please note this is representative of my personal experience the day of pre-op, and yours may be different.

How did you feel the day of the pre-op appointment? What concerned you the most? What were you told to expect?

_____

_____

_____

_____

_____

_____

_____

_____

_____

_____

_____

_____

_____

_____

5 It's Showtime

My thoughts the morning of? Calm at first. Things changed as the day progressed. The night before the big day my cousin Red stayed over so she could be with me at the hospital while we waited. When I woke up, I felt a sense of peace, and I knew that things would be okay. We all got dressed and I remember taking a photo of myself, Wayne, and our pup Shadow! I needed a physical memory of what this morning looked like, because I didn't know how the day was going to end. All of the faith in the world could not erase any of the scary thoughts of what could happen during surgery, but I left it in God's hands, and we headed to the hospital.

We had to be there at 5 am. Some family members had started to arrive because they wanted to see Wayne and Rina before they went into surgery. We were thankful to have so much love around us. I'll never forget how shaken up my mom was because she didn't think she would arrive in time to see Wayne before he went down to the operating room. Luckily, she made it. When it was time for Wayne to get prepped to head down to the holding area, I still remember the look on his face after we told each other we loved each other, and that God would get him through this. He said, "Baby I'm Scared." Seeing him scared like that did something to me and thankfully I made it to the bathroom in time before I completely lost it. I cried my heart out because he was scared, which made me sad. Yes, I was scared that my husband, my best friend, my love, my partner in crime was getting ready to have a life changing procedure, but I was faithful that it was for the best and he would live a better life afterwards. There was no way I could imagine what was going through his head. He was the one getting ready to get cut open for upwards of 6-7 hours and not know what was going to happen. He later told me that before he went under, he told himself that he was either going to wake up and see the family at the hospital or wake up and see his family in heaven. Imagine that!

The next few hours were slow. I remember clock watching and trying to figure out exactly what was going on with both Wayne and Rina during surgery. We started receiving updates about Rina first and it put my mind at ease knowing things were on track. I was able to go back and forth between the kitchen area and the waiting room talking to all of the friends and family that were there waiting with me. A new friend I had met in the transplant community came down and sat with us and helped to calm the atmosphere. She had donated to her father a while back and wanted to be there for us and be able to answer any questions the family had and offer her genuine support.

Towards the mid-afternoon we were receiving updates on Wayne about every two hours. Mentally I was fine knowing things were going well after receiving each update until about 5:30, the woman at the front desk told us that the doctor was ready to talk to us. My heart dropped as I looked at the clock. I thought something happened, because we were told he would not be finished until about 6 or 7. I remember going into a small room with his mom and sisters where we waited for the surgeon. We held hands and we prayed.

When the doctor came in, I was terrified at what was coming next. Whatever words came out of his mouth would shape how life would be. When he told us everything went well and the other surgeon was currently working on closing him back up, I dropped to my knees in praise and bawled my eyes out again. I thanked the surgeon and told him I wish I would've asked him to take pictures of the old liver and he told me he had pictures that he would send me. He did show them to me before he left the room. When I saw the pictures, I bawled again because I knew what a normal liver looked like. What I was looking at did not even seem real. I didn't ask at the time, nor will I ever ask, but based on the look of the liver they removed, I wonder how much time he really had left. But God!

The rest of the afternoon went pretty smoothly and a few hours later he was moved to the ICU where he would spend at least the next day or so. We were able to go into the room and see him, but of course he was still out of it. I was happy to be able to at least hold his hand and talk to him. His mom and I took shifts with his sisters. After some time, I had to leave the room because seeing him hooked up to all of those machines was a lot to take in, and I needed a moment to process it all.

It was about midnight when he started to wake up. The first thing he asked for was "his wife" and also for a ham sandwich. I took this as a sign that he would be just fine!

After transplant Wayne was in the hospital for nine full days. Yes, I stayed every single night except right before he was being discharged home. Arrangements had to be made to take care of the pup and when I did leave, it wasn't until someone came to visit and I was gone no longer than two hours. I needed to be present to see for myself that everything was going as expected, every step of the way. I needed to be his advocate and ensure there were no mishaps. I witnessed one of the most horrific scenes while there. His Nasogastric (NG) tube was removed and later had to be put back in while he was wide awake. I am not sure what was worse, the night when he was choking and thought he was going to die from the tube being in or the fear and pain he was in while getting the tube put back in. Both incidents were horrific, and I wouldn't wish them on anyone. The one word I could use to describe it was a wife's worst nightmare: Helplessness. There goes that word again.

The one thing that brought me comfort each night was listening to the Doppler machine that allowed us to hear the blood flowing through the liver. They tried to turn it off, but I told them no. It brought me peace and put me at ease knowing that I could actually hear the liver working. The sound was relaxing and reminded me of calm ocean waves. Nights were long because I remember asking him what seemed like every few minutes if he was okay. As long as he was okay, I was okay!

During Wayne's hospital stay a few outside stressors happened. My grandfather was in the hospital getting emergency brain surgery and one of my friend's parents was sick. I had never experienced so many feelings of stress and anxiety at one time. Let alone so much that I had absolutely no control over. I was able to sneak in about a twenty-minute visit with my grandfather before rushing right back to the hospital to be with Wayne. I was all over the place mentally, but I stayed strong the best way I knew how at the time.

There was one night towards the end of the stay, maybe day six where someone said, "I can't believe you are sleeping here every night; I couldn't do it." I remember saying, "Well I am his wife and when I became that I signed up for this. Why wouldn't I be here and where else am I supposed to be right now?" These are the hard times that test your strength as a unit, as partners. Only the strong survive.

During the nine day stay, each day had the same goal: Get up and move! Seeing him progress from moving from ICU to working with physical therapy the next day and standing was like a miracle. Each day after that the goal was to move a little more. Some days were slower than others but eventually, he was zooming around the hospital halls and walking the stairs. Rina was discharged a few days prior to Wayne but we were able to sneak in a few visits with her before she was able to go home. She was about four rooms down from Wayne and I couldn't help but go check on her and make sure she didn't need anything, because let's face it she just gave us LIFE!

A few days before discharge Wayne, his mom, and his siblings strongly urged me to go home and get a good night's sleep before he came home. He told me he was FINE and that he wanted me to get some real rest. I didn't want to go home, but I listened. Once there I realized I definitely needed that time alone! I remember going into my "she" space and allowing myself to FEEL every single emotion that was inside for who knows how long. I prayed, I cried, and I sat in silence for about 15 minutes. I slept great that night and was ready for the next part of the recovery journey.

Describe the day of transplant and post-op hospitalization. Did you have a living donor or a cadaveric donor? What was going through your mind? What was the experience like and how did you manage?

_____

_____

_____

_____

_____

_____

_____

_____

_____

_____

_____

_____

_____

_____

_____

_____

_____

_____

_____

_____

_____

_____

_____

_____

_____

_____

_____

_____

_____

_____

_____

_____

_____

_____

_____

_____

_____

_____

_____

_____

_____

_____

_____

_____

_____

_____

_____

_____

_____

_____

_____

_____

_____

_____

_____

_____

_____

_____

_____

_____

_____

_____

_____

_____

_____

_____

_____

_____

_____

_____

6 We Made It

Prior to transplant I had no idea what to expect for the post-transplant journey. I was mentally prepared to be told we needed to have home health care as well as a hospital bed for Wayne. I had thoughts of being grossed out having to drain things and clean wounds, etc. All of these things terrified me, because what if I did something wrong or hurt him?

Leading up to the day of discharge, we began having meetings with the pharmacist to learn about his medications. I was keeping track of what they were giving him daily and trying to learn the names of the meds, the dosages, as well as the purpose of them. This was so important because these meds would keep him alive and well and there was no way I could mess this up. On the day of discharge, they handed me a bag of eight different medications, which equated to him having to take more than twenty physical pills each day. To keep me sane with this I ordered a useful pill case from Amazon to keep each day organized. I was feeling ready!

We got home and nope we didn't need a hospital bed or all the other things I thought we would need. I tend to be dramatic at times....... okay a lot of the time, but I just wanted to be extra prepared since we didn't know what to expect. Wayne was situated downstairs in his man-cave for most of his recovery the first week. He slept a lot. I remember taking his temperature often and really not taking my eyes off of him. I didn't have the Doppler machine anymore to give me an audible sign that the liver was working properly. This drove me insane, but I leaned on faith to know everything was working just fine! We had home health care come in once but discharged them almost immediately because outside of asking questions, taking temps and asking about medications, there was nothing further they had to do, thank goodness! I was a nervous wreck inside but was so thankful and happy to have him home! It was time to take this journey one day at a time.

I did end up having to change one of his dressings. He was sent home with only one tube. Hallelujah! He had two or three small tubes coming out of one space that needed to be changed daily. They were extremely small and fragile, so we had to be sure not to get the medical tape on them so they would not snap. Luckily there wasn't much drainage over time, and eventually he even started wanting to do it himself.

My days looked like waking up at about 4:45-5 am daily and getting breakfast ready in time for him to take his first dose of medication at 6 am. I feel like for the first few weeks nothing mattered except for what time it was because there were certain medications that needed to be taken every twelve hours, but some couldn't be taken within two hours of another. It was a lot of management and getting used to the schedule, but it soon became second nature. I actually enjoyed when it was time to refill the medication because it was a reminder that 1. God kept him here 2. This was helping him get and stay healthy for the long haul! One important thing I would like to remind you of is to really pay attention to the side effects of the medicines, so you know what to expect. I was aware that one of his medications could potentially cause vivid dreams, so in the beginning when he started talking in his sleep and having odd dreams, I was not alarmed. These dreams were sporadic and went away after a few months. You may also experience changes in your loved one's mood and levels of empathy/compassion at times, especially if they are on any steroids. Overall it has been a pleasant post-transplant experience because he has a much more positive outlook on life now.

Ironically, the biggest adjustment I had to make post-transplant was getting used to Wayne's new appetite! He started eating things that he didn't care for prior to the transplant and started disliking things that he once loved. For instance, he used to absolutely LOVE cereal, spaghetti, and chili. He did not like pancakes, really wasn't a fan of chocolate, hated pretzels, and salmon; just to name a few. Now it is the opposite. Dinnertime conversations are so different now because where I used to be able to just cook what I knew he liked, I find myself asking, "Hey, do you still eat _____?" It drives me crazy, but it is hilarious at the same time. I learned that there is such a thing as cell memory and he has taken on some of the things that Rina loves, hence the pancakes and chocolate. Keep this in mind after your loved one's transplant. Make sure to bring up changes to the physician so they can explain what may be going on.

A month after transplant we were able to continue our tradition of hosting Thanksgiving dinner at our home. What a great way to celebrate! The only thing different that year was that Wayne was unable to pick up my mom (I did), so she could come help me cook because he was not allowed to drive yet — which if you know us well, him not being able to drive was devastating to him, but music to my ears because he has a lead foot at times.

Another thing that happened around this time was an interview with our local Channel 4 WTAE news. They came to the house prior to Thanksgiving and did a story on Wayne and Rina and it was released the week of Thanksgiving! I was so excited because people would now hear about their successful journey and hopefully give hope and encouragement to anyone else going through something similar! It also showed that there are still good people in the world with big hearts. This was the first of many interviews that occurred, and we eventually began to travel to speak at various events with the first being one of the same workshops we had attended at the beginning of our journey. We all spoke on our roles in this — donor, recipient, and wife/caregiver. Remember that visualization activity I mentioned in a previous chapter? It manifested. We were now in the middle of the post-transplant journey! We made it and could now begin to go back to some sort of normalcy and also share the testimony of what happened.

Looking back at old pictures we are now able to see how sick he really was. Prior to his health declining, Wayne was over 200lbs. Pre-Transplant he had gone down to about 173 and by the time he was discharged home and started losing all the fluid he had gained while inpatient, he had gone down to 158lbs! I noticed changes in his weight along the way but didn't notice the transformation until I saw pictures to compare. His weight or physical changes were never something that affected me because in sickness and in health — he means the world to me.

I was blessed to be able to be out of work for six weeks on paid FMLA. I went back to work after Thanksgiving. Wayne was out a little longer of course and returned back to work on January 29, 2019. Rina had gone back to work about two weeks after she was discharged. It still blows my mind that I am able to look back on this entire experience as a memory. When it was just an idea, it was something I could not even imagine going through, something I know we both never wanted to have to go through, let alone actually overcoming it and talking about it in the past tense. But here we were and we made it! We had a huge surprise celebration after the one year "Liverversary." Close family and friends came from all over and we celebrated Wayne and Rina with good food and lots of laughs and love!

What was life like once your loved one was home and recovering? What were you feeling during this time? How did things change?

_____

_____

_____

_____

_____

_____

_____

_____

_____

_____

_____

_____

_____

_____

_____

_____

_____

_____

_____

_____

7 Okay, Now What?

Now that the transplant has been taken care of, it leaves the question of what now for the caregiver? I was so used to silently stressing for years on end and doing all that I could to make sure everything was okay with Wayne that I realized I had started lacking in my own self-care. When was the last time I had a physical and bloodwork done? Even though I felt okay, was I truly fine? I finally made the decision to declare 2019 as the year of Self-Care in ALL areas of my life! I made an appointment for my physical and blood work and found out that my cholesterol and blood sugar were high, so I made it my duty and priority to bring those numbers down!

Another part of my newfound self-care was to really figure out how I wanted to spend my time and what truly made me feel personally fulfilled, versus how I had been spending my time! For the first four years of our marriage, in addition to my regular 9-5 career, I was doing sales for a health and wellness company. Over those years I honestly thought I was trying to find myself, however it wasn't until after I had these six weeks out of work to really focus and think about life as a whole, I realized I had actually lost myself. I learned in this season what was truly important to me, and that was being present in the moment, spending time with my loved ones, having peace, and doing things I truly enjoyed. I decided in January 2019 to completely step away from the business I was a part of and launch my natural nail service business called Pampered Living! After receiving my cosmetology license in 2010 I had worked in spas and salons over the years, and then moved to being mobile, but I was only doing services here and there. I spent way too much time being afraid and I found that I was comparing myself to other amazing nail techs who had other skills, so I allowed myself to fall back. In this season I decided to carve out my niche, become official, and go for it and the rest of my 2019 was a success and it was just the beginning! I am glad I started putting one foot in front of the other, stepping away from what was familiar and comfortable and just going for it! I reclaimed my peace and things are going well.

So that's it! We are both back to work and getting into the swing of our new normal. There have been speaking engagements here and there, trips to living donor conferences, continued bi-weekly bloodwork, and follow up appointments, but for the most part, no more stress about when or if this disease would progress! It's gone! Now, we do still have some appointments and treatments for his ulcerative colitis, but as far as the liver disease he only has to get evaluated about every six months to a year right now. I don't think of the fact that they say transplant is a treatment and not a cure. We take each day one at a time and we are both diligent about knowing when meds need to be adjusted or when to call to ask questions about symptoms; no question is too small. This is a lifelong journey but thankfully, the hardest part is behind us now. What warms my heart is that God saw fit to keep my husband here on this earth and I cherish every day that we have together, whether good, bad or indifferent, because things could have turned out quite differently.

I am forever grateful.

It is so important to remember to take time during this journey to have a few moments to yourself. It gets stressful and you will feel like nothing else matters at times except making sure your loved one is okay. You will constantly get asked about how your loved one is doing of course and no, not many will ask how you are doing. Sometimes you say to yourself, "What about me, there were actually two journeys going on." Now, this isn't to sound selfish but unless you are a caregiver, you have no idea what the other side of the journey feels like internally. Sometimes you will suppress those feelings, not wanting to feel or sound selfish, or you will tell yourself that this wasn't about you, so you have no right to have these feelings. However, your feelings are valid. You are in this together and I want you to know that you must not feel bad if you decide you need a few hours or even a day to yourself. If someone offers you help, don't feel badly about accepting it. You have done an amazing job at caring for your loved one and doing the absolute BEST that you can during this uncertain journey! We were blessed to have the outcome that we did. You are phenomenal and though everyone's story will be different, the steps in the journey are quite similar! Please know that you are not alone in this; we are our own community who understands what the other is going through, went through, or will go through! Your life may turn out for the better or some cases may not. Know that nothing is your fault; you are only human and can only do what is in your scope. Do NOT beat yourself up about anything and don't be so hard on yourself. Do not lose yourself during the journey. Most importantly, be sure to keep up with your own doctor's appointments during this time.

Please utilize the self-care suggestion list at the end of this journal to remind yourself to do something for you from time to time. I've also included a medication tracker, a bloodwork tracker, as well as space to document the Initial, Pre, and Post-operative office visits. Keeping yourself organized will be extremely important during this time. It is my hope that you are able to utilize this journal to document your feelings and experience and organize your loved one's care. I appreciate you for taking the time to read about our journey and want to tell you that your story will also inspire others. Never be afraid to share it.

Use the space below to reflect on yourself and anything you discovered about yourself during your caregiving journey. What changes did you make within yourself? What are you looking forward to?

_____

_____

_____

_____

_____

_____

_____

_____

_____

_____

_____

_____

_____

_____

_____

_____

_____

_____

_____

_____

_____

_____

_____

_____

_____

_____

_____

_____

_____

_____

_____

_____

_____

_____

_____

_____

_____

_____

_____

_____

_____

_____

_____

_____

_____

_____

_____

_____

_____

_____

_____

_____

_____

_____

_____

_____

100 Self-Care Ideas

1. Write in your journal.

2. Pray.

3. Take a long hot shower.

4. Let out that cry you've been holding onto.

5. Take a nature walk.

6. Read a book.

7. Sleep in a little longer than usual.

8. Get or give yourself a manicure or pedicure.

9. Cook your favorite meal.

10. Eat a cookie and do not feel guilty.

11. Listen to music.

12. Blast music while you clean the house.

13. Sit outside and enjoy the breeze.

14. Take a nap.

15. Go shopping.

16. Put your phone on do not disturb for a few hours.

17. Look through old photo albums.

18. Clear out your emails.

19. Organize the photos on your phone.

20. Meditate.

21. Try a new fitness activity.

22. No social media for 24 hours

23. Do a liquid fast for 24 hours.

24. Try a new recipe.

25. Give yourself an organic facial.

26. Get a massage.

27. Look at houses online.

28. Read a magazine.

29. Drink a glass of wine.

30. Go to a pet store or animal shelter.

31. Go for a drive with the windows down.

32. Create a relaxing space in your home just for you.

33. Walk around the mall.

34. Go and get ice cream.

35. Purge your closet.

36. Donate unwanted items.

37. Pay it forward in a drive thru.

38. Plan a short weekend get-away.

39. Make your own annual doctor's appointments.

40. Say yes when people offer to help you if you need it.

41. Say no to things you don't want to do.

42. Drink at least 64oz of water per day.

43. Have a karaoke session at home.

44. Light your favorite candles.

45. Watch old family videos.

46. Start a project on which you've been procrastinating.

47. Clean your jewelry.

48. Listen to a podcast.

49. Update your resume.

50. Visit your local bakery and have a treat.

51. Listen to soft jazz music to relax.

52. Organize your spice cabinet.

53. Have a backyard picnic.

54. Have breakfast for dinner.

55. Make S'mores, the normal way or in the air fryer.

56. Join a support group.

57. Call a friend and talk on the phone for hours.

58. Write a poem.

59. Record a voice message to yourself of your feelings.

60. Learn a new dance.

61. Get at least 30min of cardio every day.

62. Speak positive affirmations daily.

63. Listen to something motivational every day.

64. Dream out loud - Plan your dream home or vacation.

65. Organize your important papers.

66. Know that it's okay not to be okay 24/7.

67. Ask for whatever help you've needed.

68. Binge watch your favorite television shows.

69. Start your business plan.

70. Roll up loose change and take it to the bank.

71. Start an at home DIY project.

72. Get into some yard work.

73. Learn how to do something new.

74. Read an actual newspaper and not online.

75. Bake cookies.

76. Get dressed and take yourself on a dinner date.

77. Organize your budget.

78. Go over your bills and eliminate unnecessary items.

79. Close your eyes and sit in silence for a few minutes.

80. Practice deep breathing exercises.

81. Create a Pinterest account.

82. Learn how to play Chess.

83. Do the one thing that scares you the most.

84. Pick a day to do absolutely NOTHING!

85. Open the windows in your home for natural light.

86. Take an interesting free online course.

87. Perfect your craft (whatever it may be).

88. Get coloring books and crayons let your creativity flow.

89. Window-shop online.

90. Re-arrange a room in your house to create a new vibe.

91. Put your laundry away immediately after it dries.

92. Make your own exfoliating lip or body scrub.

93. Go thrift shopping.

94. Practice the law of attraction and positive thinking.

95. Drink a soothing hot cup of tea. Biscotti optional!

96. Ride your bike around the block.

97. Watch a comedy show on Netflix.

98. Paint a room in your house.

99. Add a bunch of items to your Amazon wish list for later.

100. Take a trip down memory lane with your loved ones and share funny stories.

MEDICATION TRACKER

Date Prescribed	Medication Type	Dosage AM/PM	Frequency per Week	What Time to Take Meds

Date Prescribed	Medication Type	Dosage AM/PM	Frequency per Week	What Time to Take Meds

Date Prescribed	Medication Type	Dosage AM/PM	Frequency per Week	What Time to Take Meds

Date Prescribed	Medication Type	Dosage AM/PM	Frequency per Week	What Time to Take Meds

Date Prescribed	Medication Type	Dosage AM/PM	Frequency per Week	What Time to Take Meds

Date Prescribed	Medication Type	Dosage AM/PM	Frequency per Week	What Time to Take Meds

Date Prescribed	Medication Type	Dosage AM/PM	Frequency per Week	What Time to Take Meds

Date Prescribed	Medication Type	Dosage AM/PM	Frequency per Week	What Time to Take Meds

Date Prescribed	Medication Type	Dosage AM/PM	Frequency per Week	What Time to Take Meds

Date Prescribed	Medication Type	Dosage AM/PM	Frequency per Week	What Time to Take Meds

BLOODWORK TRACKER

Date Blood Was Drawn	Levels Elevated Yes or No	Medication Adjusted	Medication Name	New Dosage

Date Blood Was Drawn	Levels Elevated Yes or No	Medication Adjusted	Medication Name	New Dosage

Date Blood Was Drawn	Levels Elevated Yes or No	Medication Adjusted	Medication Name	New Dosage

Date Blood Was Drawn	Levels Elevated Yes or No	Medication Adjusted	Medication Name	New Dosage

Date Blood Was Drawn	Levels Elevated Yes or No	Medication Adjusted	Medication Name	New Dosage

Date Blood Was Drawn	Levels Elevated Yes or No	Medication Adjusted	Medication Name	New Dosage

Date Blood Was Drawn	Levels Elevated Yes or No	Medication Adjusted	Medication Name	New Dosage

Date Blood Was Drawn	Levels Elevated Yes or No	Medication Adjusted	Medication Name	New Dosage

Date Blood Was Drawn	Levels Elevated Yes or No	Medication Adjusted	Medication Name	New Dosage

Date Blood Was Drawn	Levels Elevated Yes or No	Medication Adjusted	Medication Name	New Dosage

Appointment Notes

Initial Evaluation:

_____

_____

_____

_____

_____

_____

_____

_____

_____

_____

_____

_____

_____

_____

_____

_____

_____

_____

_____

_____

_____

_____

_____

_____

_____

_____

_____

_____

_____

_____

_____

_____

_____

_____

_____

_____

_____

_____

_____

_____

_____

_____

_____

_____

Pre-Operative Notes:

Post-Operative Notes:

_____

_____

_____

_____

_____

_____

_____

_____

_____

_____

_____

_____

_____

_____

_____

_____

_____

_____

_____

_____

Acknowledgements

I would first like to thank God for putting this project on my heart and giving me the discipline to complete it. This is for the next person who will need some encouragement in knowing they are not alone!

Rina Kader - our angel, our sister THANK YOU! It is because of your selfless, altruistic act of kindness that this journey turned out the way that it did. We can't thank you enough. You are a part of our family now. Literally! LOL!

Wayne - You always did what you had to do during this process. You never missed a doctor's appointment and stayed on top of your health the entire time. I admire you for never giving up! We've made it through so much over the years and I am glad God saw fit for me to be the one to take this journey with you! I love you more than you know!

I would like to thank the staff of the UPMC Living Donor Program and the staff of the Frank Sarris Outpatient Clinic at the Thomas Starzl Transplantation Institute. Every physician, surgeon, fellow, pharmacist, nutritionist, anesthesiologist, Nurse, CNA, Housekeeper, and all of the staff of 11N at Montefiore who had a part in this journey. Specifically, Dr. Swaytha Ganesh, Dr. Abhinav Humar, & Dr. Christopher Hughes for saving my husband's life. Thank you to Donya Lee, the UPMC Living Donor Ambassador who eased my mind the first time we met. Thank you to Ms. Gladys, the supervisor of housekeeping and family friend, for ensuring Wayne and Rina's rooms were immaculate as well as for sending us food during our stay.

To those who were there the day of the transplant that made the wait much easier, and calmed my nerves: my Mom Tina Davidson, Stepdad Poppy, Aunt Tammy, Aunt Staci, Uncle Mike, Brandon Green, Ray Nell Jones for being there almost daily, Diana McDonald for sharing your journey, and staying with us almost the entire time that day, Aunt Janice, Cousin Nikki, Cousin Valerie, Cousin Marla, My momma #2 - Ms. Laureen, Father-In-Law - Wayne Sr., Sister Shawnee, Sister Kisha, Uncle Kenny, Aunt Velma, Cousin Red, and Brotha Mike! Thank you to my neighbor family, The Banners, for coming to visit. Thank you, Terri and Monica, for Cash-Apping me to purchase lunch on the days I stayed at the hospital. To my grandparents Fay and Robert for offering words of encouragement even while my grandad was inpatient going through his own health issues. Thank you to my dad Edward Perkins, my Stepmom Arlene Perkins, and my sisters Arnette Webb and Michelle Harper for the support from afar! Thank you to my cousin Anntoinette Sweeting for sending the amazing get well gift. Thank you to my girls for being there for us in spirit during that time; Amber, Angel, Shawnda, Sierra, Norma, and Danielle. Even with distance, the love was, and is always felt!

To each and every cousin, uncle, aunt, and friend of mine and/or Wayne's who text, called, visited, prayed, shared a social media post, or got evaluated initially – We love and appreciate you! To our 'nurse cousins' Shayla and Kamara – thank you for always being there for me when I have questions or need a facetime walk through on how to administer an injection. To my career/life mentor and friend Virginia, thank God for you! To Nicole, Kia, Yo, and Nickia; my accountability partners during the creation of this journal – I appreciate you!

I was at a networking happy hour in early 2019 and a woman I am connected to on Facebook named Darcel Madkins, asked me when the book was coming out. I looked at her thinking to myself "What are you talking about?" She said, "Well the chapters are already written." I put this in the back of my mind because I had not heard this from God yet and I had no intention of writing a book. Over time, I participated in a few conversations in a Facebook caregiver group and offered encouragement or shared my journey, and also felt like people were having difficulty understanding how I was feeling as anniversary dates of different parts of the journey came up. I started to hear more clearly from God that I was not alone in this, and that I needed to create a journal for everyone else feeling like they needed an outlet. At that moment, the creation of this journal began.

I pray it is as therapeutic for you reading and writing in this journal, as it was for me creating it.

About the Author

Tasha Livingston was born and raised in Pittsburgh, Pennsylvania. She obtained her Bachelor of Science in Business Administration from the University of Pittsburgh. Her passions include traveling, spending time with family, and all things self-care. She is the Owner and Operator of a mobile natural nail service called Pampered Living. She is a devoted wife to her husband Wayne who is a Living Donor Liver Transplant recipient as of October 22, 2018. She is also a dog mom to a rambunctious German shepherd named "Shadow." This is her first writing project, and it was conceptualized and written out of passion and necessity for "Those Who Care!"

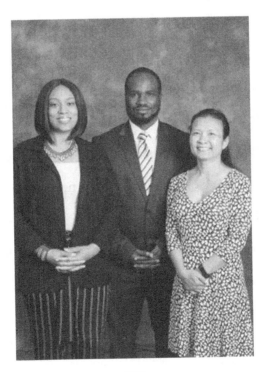

Contact information:

Email: thosewhocarejourney@gmail.com

Facebook: Those Who Care Journey

Instagram: @thosewhocarejourney

Website: http://thosewhocarejourney.com